Physical Therapy Aide:
What You Need to Know

Contents

Introduction

First off, I want to congratulate you on picking this book up and making an effort to better yourself as a physical therapy aide. This book will serve as a guide for those just starting out with no experience and for those who have been working as an aide and want to master their skills. If you feel that you have benefited at all from the knowledge shared in this book, please leave a 5-star review. This will help spread the information to current and future physical therapy aides.

For most of you, choosing to pursue a position as a physical therapy aide is your first exposure to healthcare. I want to personally welcome you into the exciting and rewarding field of rehabilitation services. This guide will teach you everything you need to know to be the physical therapy aide that therapists want.

Working as an aide, it took me months to master every component of the physical therapy clinic. I decided to create this guide so you can learn from my struggles. This will shorten your learning curve so you can master your position in no time!

Speaking with several Physical Therapists from every area of Physical Therapy, I was able to create a guide with the most pertinent information that therapists wished their aides would master quickly.

I have worked in outpatient private practice, cardiac rehab, and inpatient rehab. I have accumulated roughly 6 years of physical therapy aide experience before I attended Physical Therapy school.

This book is structured so that the facts and information that you need to know are listed first and the clinical skills, which you can only master with repetition, are described after.

Once again congratulations on taking this step to better yourself, learn about the world of physical therapy, and to most importantly impress your employer with the knowledge that you will acquire in the following chapters.

What is a Physical Therapy Aide?

A physical therapy aide is an unlicensed member of the physical therapy clinic who assists the therapists with the treatment plan of a patient. A physical therapy aide is NOT a physical therapy assistant (PTA). A PTA has formal education and a license to practice under a physical therapist.

The aide acts as an extra set of hands wherever needed. Common duties include giving ice and hot packs to patients when needed, applying electrical stimulation, perform ultrasounds, help patients get on and off equipment, help guide and correct patients through their therapeutic exercise programs, and maintenance of the therapy area. An aide cannot provide any sort of treatment on the patient that is not approved by the therapist and can never provide any sort of manual therapy. As an aide, you are a key component in keeping the flow of patients so they can receive proper care from the therapist, which will consequently improve the patient experience.

Non patient-related tasks of an aide could include housekeeping, administrative, and clerical duties.

How to be Extraordinary

This is your time to impress and create healthy relationships with the therapists. Since most of you will need letters from professional references, it is important to go above and beyond your basic duties in order to receive positive letters of recommendations. Think of the time and energy that you put into your role as an investment for the future. The more you contribute to the functioning of the Physical therapy unit, the higher return you will receive. In this case, the return would be the recommendations that will set you apart from all the other applicants.

First, the most important way to be extraordinary is making the therapist's life easier. You can do this by anticipating the needs of the therapist before they ask. It takes some time to get used to the way each therapist operates. Being observant from your first shift as an aide will help shorten your learning curve on what the therapist needs and when they need it.

Second, be able to prioritize your tasks efficiently. You have many responsibilities and it is your job to judge which task is most important. For example, your duties will most likely include cleaning tables and folding laundry. Since your main responsibility is to maintain the flow of the clinic, it is more important to clean off a table when someone is done with treatment in order to open it up for the next patient than it is to fold laundry. Laundry in the clinic is important and ultimately needs to be done, but maintaining patient flow is most important.

Third, multi-tasking and time management skills must be optimal. The patient always comes first. At times you will have multiple patients to take care of. One example is if you are working with two patients. Patient A has to do a short exercise, bike for 10 minutes, then needs ice once they are done. Patient B needs an ultrasound and then ice after. The most efficient way to handle this scenario would be to guide Patient A through their short exercise. While they are doing that, you go setup Patient B for their ultrasound. Once Patient B is setup, Patient A will have just finished with their exercise. Put Patient A on the bike and that will give you a 10 minute window in order to ultrasound Patient B and get them on ice. By the time Patient B is situated and on ice, Patient A would just have finished with the bike and be ready for ice in which you can provide them with

right away since you managed your time

effectively with multi-tasking. This is important

to the patient flow and experience because both

patients will have received optimal care while

not having to wait around for you to be available.

Types of Settings

1. Outpatient Orthopedics

If you like solving problems and working with an active population, you'll probably love outpatient orthopedics. There are many differences within outpatient ortho, though. Some clinics largely treat active older adults, while others specialize in working with athletes, teens, or even primarily post-operative patient loads.

Different clinics have different business models. Some see follow-up patients every 15 minutes and others may see them for 30 minute sessions.

Your task duties may differ depending on where you work as an aide. For example, with many larger public health systems such as UCLA, aides are absolutely unable to perform ultrasound or set up electrical stimulations. However, in many private practices, the therapists allow the aides to perform some of these modalities. The consequence is that the providing therapist risks their licensure whenever they allow you to participate in a treatment.

2. Inpatient

Some PTs assert that inpatient rehabilitation is the purest form of physical therapy there is, because patients typically make enormous functional gains in a brief, intensive time period. Most patients spend 2-3 weeks in inpatient rehab, and they're seen by multiple therapy disciplines.

Inpatient rehab patients have often suffered strokes, traumatic brain injuries, or serious accidents that have impaired their ability to walk, dress themselves, feed themselves, and (sometimes) even speak.

As an aide for inpatient, your main responsibilities include assisting the the PT with bed mobility and some gait training.

3. Acute Care

Acute care is a fancy way of saying "the hospital," and PTs who work in acute care tend to see all sorts of illnesses and injuries, from a debilitating case of pneumonia that leaves a patient too weak to get out of bed, to a traumatic accident that leaves a patient without a limb. This setting is exciting and collaborative, and by shadowing in acute care, you'll get to witness PTs working alongside physicians, nurses, occupational therapists, speech language pathologists, respiratory therapists, and other medical professionals. Acute care PTs tend to see patients for only a few days at a time, which is unlike most other practice settings, where patients might be seen for many days or weeks—or even months—on end.

4. Skilled Nursing Facility

Also known as a nursing home or a long-term care facility, a skilled nursing facility (SNF) is a building (or group of buildings) with round-the-clock nursing care, as well as rehabilitation services.

SNFs house patients who are unable to care for themselves for both the short-term and the long-term. PTs who work in SNFs will evaluate and assess these patients, determining whether their functional mobility levels have declined from their baseline levels. If the patients are deemed below their functional baseline, the PTs will work with them to improve their sitting, standing, and walking abilities.

5. Home Health

Home health physical therapy is an extremely unique and rewarding setting, and therapists enjoy quite a bit of flexibility and autonomy in this setting. Home health PTs visit patients in their homes and provide extremely functional treatments that utilize patients' own furniture and equipment. PTs working in this setting also make home safety recommendations, perform caregiver education, and provide training on everything from equipment transfers to conserving energy while cooking or performing hygiene.

The use of aides in this setting are rare, maybe nonexistent, but still good to know about.

<u>Modalities</u>

As an aide you will more than likely be asked to provide modalities for the patients to help with their therapy. Modalities are instruments physical therapists utilize to either increase or decrease circulation to an area or to create a pain gating effect. Pain gating refers to stimulus applied in the attempts to interrupt the nerve impulse signaling pain to the brain. Touch sensation travels through thicker nerve fibers where pain is sent through smaller nerve fibers; thus, the stimulus from touch inundates the brain more quickly decreasing the brains response to pain stimulus. These modalities can include cryotherapy, thermotherapy, ultrasound, and different types of electrical stimulation.

*Note: The ultrasound and electrical stimulation machines should not be used on pregnant women, patients with tumors (malignant or benign), through the eyeball or carotid sinus, or on individuals with pace makers. *

Ice

Ice packs are used to both decrease circulation and pain responses superficially. It should be applied anywhere from 10 to 20 minutes but no longer. If ice is left on greater than 20 minutes, you get a rebound of circulation to the area resulting in a return of edema. You must use precaution when placing ice packs directly on the skin of children or the elderly. Their decreased sensitivity of their skin makes them prone to frost nip.

Heat

Moist heat packs are used to increase circulation superficially, increase tissue pliability and flexibility, as well as decrease pain. Heat should be applied for approximately 10 minutes. Extra layers should be used with children and the elderly due to the generalized decreased sensitivity and decreased ability to dissipate heat. Furthermore, you should not heat a pregnant woman's back or abdomen to prevent thermal change in the womb.

Ultrasound

Ultrasound is a machine that translates electricity into sound waves for deeper circulatory changes in soft tissues such as muscles, tendons, and ligaments. The ultrasound provides a thermal/heating effect for increased tissue healing and pliability. Pulsed parameters of the machine are used for flushing inflammation or a phonophoresis which is the transcutaneous delivery of medication. There must be ultrasound gel or water between the sound head and the body in order for the sound waves to conduct. Without this substance, the crystals in the sound head can be permanently damaged or could burn a patient. Ultrasound should never be performed over an eye or a pregnant woman's uterus/back due to the presence of vital fluids in these cavities.

H-Wave

H-Wave is an electrical stimulation unit used to increase circulation, thus increasing healing rate. There is a low frequency parameter that should be set when you first see a small contraction of the motor units under the electrodes. There is a high frequency setting that should be set as high as the patient is comfortable tolerating in order to create a pain gating effect. It too increases circulation to the area applied, thus increasing the healing rate.

H-Wave has a set protocol designated in the book provided with the machine. The representatives highly encourage health care professionals to stick with the parameters suggested for maximum benefits. However, variations of these parameters have proven effective. Alterations to the time frames, placement of the electrodes, or the inclusion of

cryotherapy with the high frequency setting is

used when the PT is primarily looking for pain

gating effect (not increased circulation).

Interferential

Interferential stimulation (commonly referred to as IFC) is another electrical stimulation unit that works primarily for decreasing edema in joint spaces. These electrodes must be placed surrounding the joint space you want to effect and the channels must be crisscrossed. This unit will not be effective if the channels are parallel to one another. The waves from the two channels travel at different rates and summate where they intersect. This is the place that is truly impacted by the IFC unit (not where the actual electrodes are located). Ice is often used at the same time for a more affective treatment. This unit should not be combined with thermal agents.

TENS

TENS is a Transcutaneous Electrical Nerve Stimulator and is used for pain gating only. It can be used to journal pain responses over time. The TENS unit can be used continuously over a long time as long as the patient is changing the stimulus setting every few days to avoid accommodation of the nervous system to the same stimulus.

MENS

MENS is a Microcurrent Electrical Neuromuscular Stimulator for the treatment of acute or chronic pain. Research has shown that injured tissues generate electrical currents that differ from those of healthy cells. The MENS inputs an artificial external electrical current that is similar to the body's physiological electrical current for homeostasis and tissue healing. This unit can be used for a wide variety of treatments and check with the therapist to see which settings would be useful. Most settings are termed sub-sensory. However, some acute pain patients will reach their threshold more quickly than chronic pain patients. Probe setting needs to be held until 100% conductivity is measured which is typically a matter of seconds. The probes must be saturated with water and the wet tip must touch the metal base in order for this setting to work. All other settings require electrodes to be placed and are recommended to be on for 20-30 minutes.

NMES

Neuromuscular Electrical Stimulation unit (NMES) is placed on weak /atrophied muscles to stimulate a muscle contraction during exercises for hypertrophy and proper timing. This unit must be placed on the muscle and turned up while the patient is relaxed so you can see the electrically stimulated contraction before the patient can start contracting actively with the unit. This modality is picked up by the sensory nerves before you will see the motor units contract; so turn the dial up slowly while monitoring the patient's tolerance until you see the full contraction (tetanus) of the targeted muscle.

Cervical and Lumbar Traction:

Traction is used to decompress the discs of the vertebral column. During the day the vertebral discs compress due to gravity. This creates pressure on the discs which make them more susceptible to injury or increase pain and discomfort in patients with current spinal disorders. This procedure can help restore neurological function in limbs and temporarily relieve discomfort associated with pressure on the discs.

There are two types of traction, cervical and lumbar. Cervical traction decompresses the discs of the neck and lumbar traction decompresses the discs of the lower back.

Usually the therapist will set up the patient on these modalities. Therapists will normally allow you to take the patient off traction but ask for

permission before.

Anatomy

Working in physical therapy requires knowledge of anatomy and anatomical movements and positions. Here is a list of relevant anatomy that you will need to master.

Anatomical directions

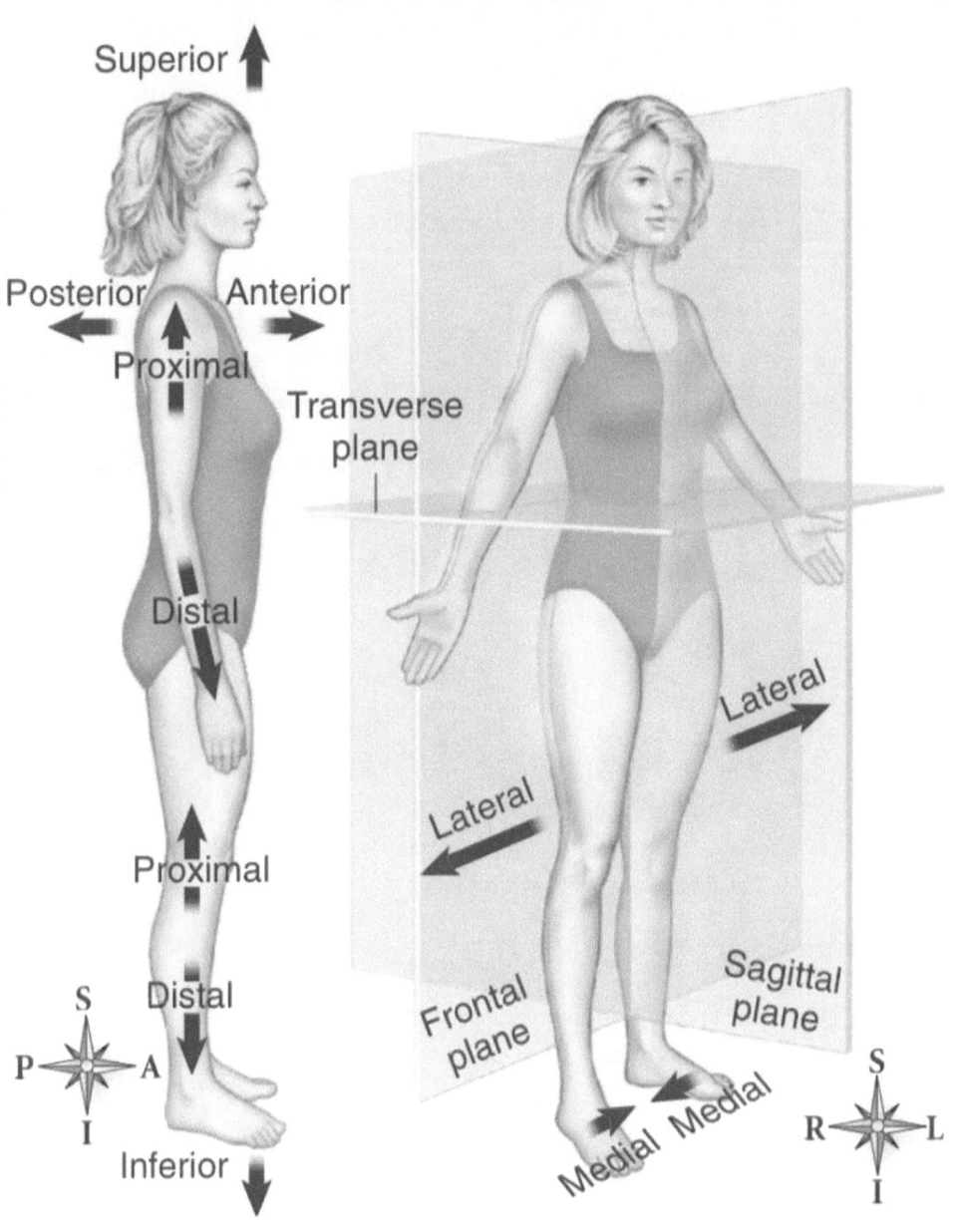

✳ TABLE 1-27   Anatomic Directions Listed in Opposite Pairs

Directional Term	Definition	Example of Use
Left	To the left of the body or structure being studied (not *your* left, the subject's)	The stomach is to the *left* of the liver.
Right	To the right of the body or structure being studied	The *right* kidney is damaged.
Lateral	Toward the side; away from the midsagittal plane	The eyes are *lateral* to the nose.
Medial	Toward the midsagittal plane; away from the side	The eyes are *medial* to the ears.
Anterior	Toward the front of the body	The nose is on the *anterior* of the head.
Posterior	Toward the back (rear) of the body	The heel is *posterior* to the head.
Superior	Toward the top of the body	The shoulders are *superior* to the hips.
Inferior	Toward the bottom of the body	The stomach is *inferior* to the heart.

* TABLE 2-4 Terms Used to Describe Bone Markings

Terms	Pronunciations	Descriptions and Translations	Examples
Angle	ANG-gul	An inside or outside corner	Angle of mandible
			Inferior angle of scapula
Body	BOD-ee	The main or central portion of a bone	Body of sphenoid bone
			Body of vertebra
			Body of sternum
			Body of rib
Condyle	KON-dyle	Rounded bump; usually fits into a fossa on another bone to form a joint (literally "knuckle")	Occipital condyle
			Lateral condyle of femur
			Medial condyle of tibia
Crest	krest	Moderately raised ridge; generally a site for muscle attachment (literally "tuft" or "comb")	Pubic crest of coxal (pelvic) bone
			Intertrochanteric crest of femur
			Crest of tibia
Epicondyle	ep-i-KON-dyle	Bump near a condyle; often gives the appearance of a "bump on a bump"; for muscle attachment (literally "upon a knuckle")	Lateral epicondyle of humerus
			Medial epicondyle of humerus
			Lateral epicondyle of femur
Foramen (pl., foramina or foramens)	foh-RAY-men or FO-ra-men (foh-RAM-in-ah or foh-RAY-menz)	Round hole for vessels and nerves (literally "hole")	Jugular foramen of temporal bone
			Foramen ovale of sphenoid bone
			Obturator foramen of coxal (pelvic) bone
Fossa (pl., fossae)	FOSS-ah (FOSS-ee)	Depression; often receives an articulating bone (literally "ditch")	Mandibular fossa of temporal bone
			Olecranon fossa of humerus
			Intercondylar fossa of femur
Head	hed	Distinct epiphysis on a long bone, separated from the shaft by a narrowed portion or neck	Head of humerus
			Head of radius
			Head of femur

Terms	Pronunciations	Descriptions and Translations	Examples
Line (Latin *linea*)	lyne (LEEN-ee-ah or LIN-ee-ah)	Similar to a crest but not raised as much (is often rather faint)	Superior nuchal line of occipital bone
			Superior temporal line of parietal bone
			Intercondylar line of femur
Neck	nek	A narrowed portion, usually at the base of a head	Neck of rib
			Neck of radius
			Neck of femur
Notch	notch	A V-like "cut" out of the margin or edge of a flat area	Supraorbital notch
			Radial notch of ulna
			Greater sciatic notch of coxal bone
Process	PRAH-ses or PRO-ses	Projection or raised area	Mastoid process of temporal bone
			Spinous process of vertebra
			Coronoid process of ulna
Sinus	SYE-nus	Cavity within a bone (literally "hollow")	Frontal sinus
			Sphenoid sinus
			Maxillary sinus
Spine	spyne	Sharp, pointed process; similar to crested but raised more; for muscle attachment (literally "thorn")	Spine of scapula
			Spine of vertebra
			Ischial spine
Tubercle	TOO-ber-kul	Small tuberosity (see below); small oblong bump (literally "small bump" or "small lump")	Tubercle of rib
			Greater tubercle of humerus
			Adductor tubercle of femur

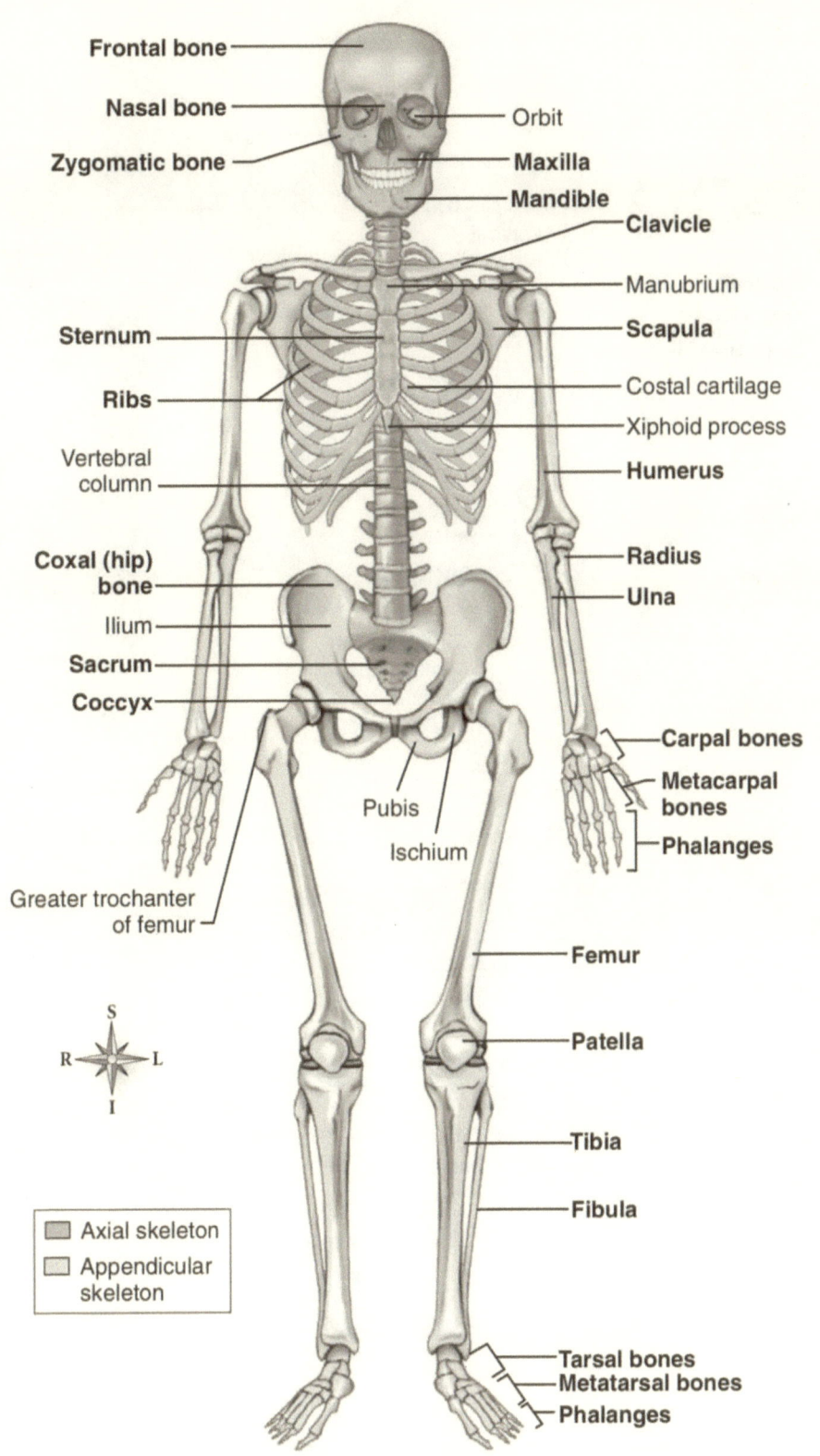

Frontal bone

Nasal bone

Zygomatic bone

Orbit

Maxilla

Mandible

Clavicle

Manubrium

Scapula

Costal cartilage

Xiphoid process

Humerus

Sternum

Ribs

Vertebral
column

**Coxal (hip)
bone**

Ilium

Sacrum

Coccyx

Radius

Ulna

Carpal bones

**Metacarpal
bones**

Phalanges

Pubis

Ischium

Greater trochanter
of femur

Femur

S

R ✹ L

I

Patella

Tibia

Fibula

☐ Axial skeleton
☐ Appendicular
   skeleton

Tarsal bones
Metatarsal bones
Phalanges

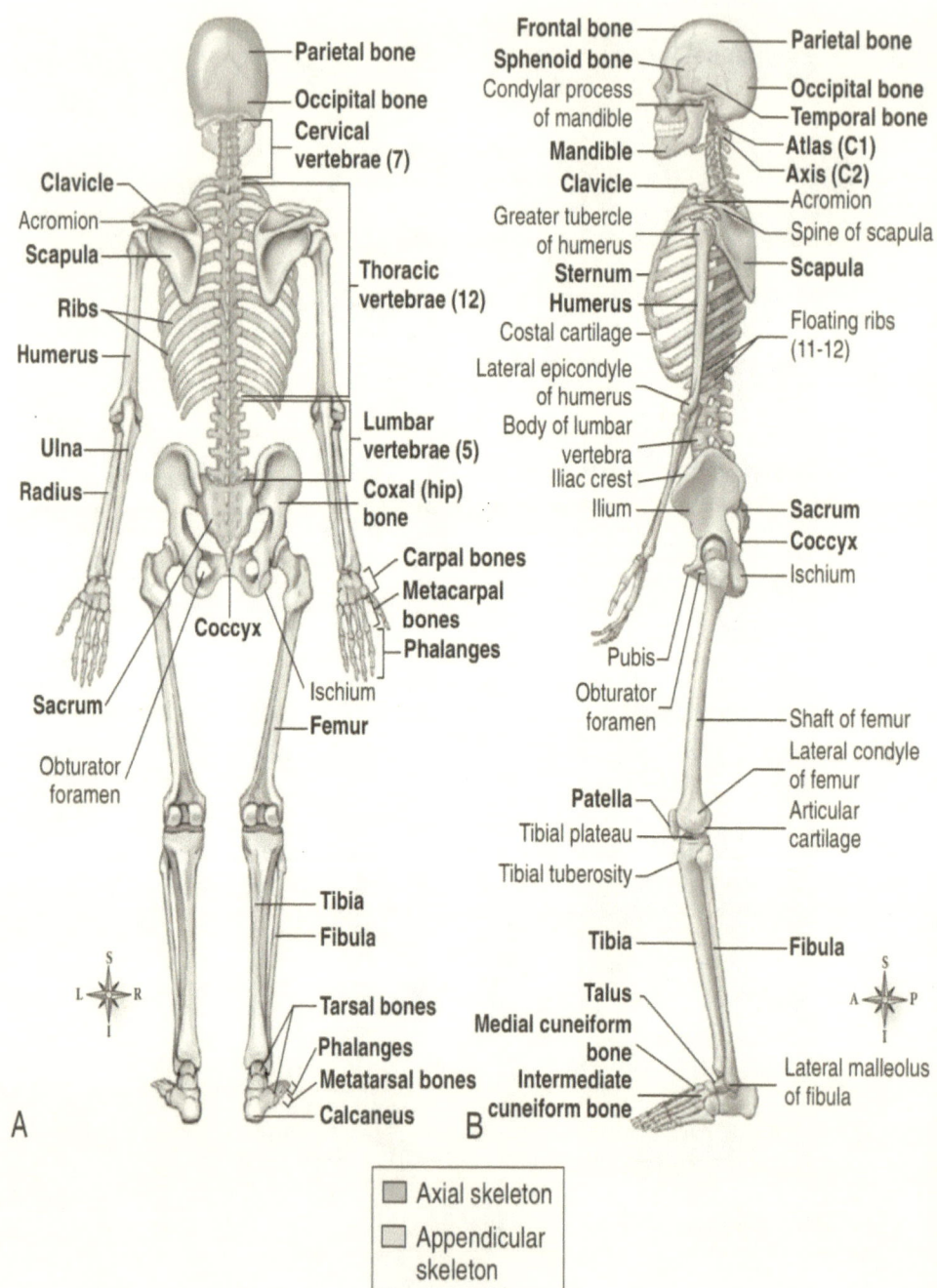

Parietal bone
Occipital bone
Cervical vertebrae (7)
Clavicle
Acromion
Scapula
Ribs
Humerus
Ulna
Radius
Thoracic vertebrae (12)
Lumbar vertebrae (5)
Coxal (hip) bone
Carpal bones
Metacarpal bones
Phalanges
Coccyx
Ischium
Sacrum
Femur
Obturator foramen
Tibia
Fibula
Tarsal bones
Phalanges
Metatarsal bones
Calcaneus

S
L R
I

A

Frontal bone
Sphenoid bone
Condylar process of mandible
Mandible
Clavicle
Greater tubercle of humerus
Sternum
Humerus
Costal cartilage
Lateral epicondyle of humerus
Body of lumbar vertebra
Iliac crest
Ilium
Pubis
Obturator foramen
Patella
Tibial plateau
Tibial tuberosity
Tibia
Talus
Medial cuneiform bone
Intermediate cuneiform bone

Parietal bone
Occipital bone
Temporal bone
Atlas (C1)
Axis (C2)
Acromion
Spine of scapula
Scapula
Floating ribs (11-12)
Sacrum
Coccyx
Ischium
Shaft of femur
Lateral condyle of femur
Articular cartilage
Fibula
Lateral malleolus of fibula

S
A P
I

B

Axial skeleton
Appendicular skeleton

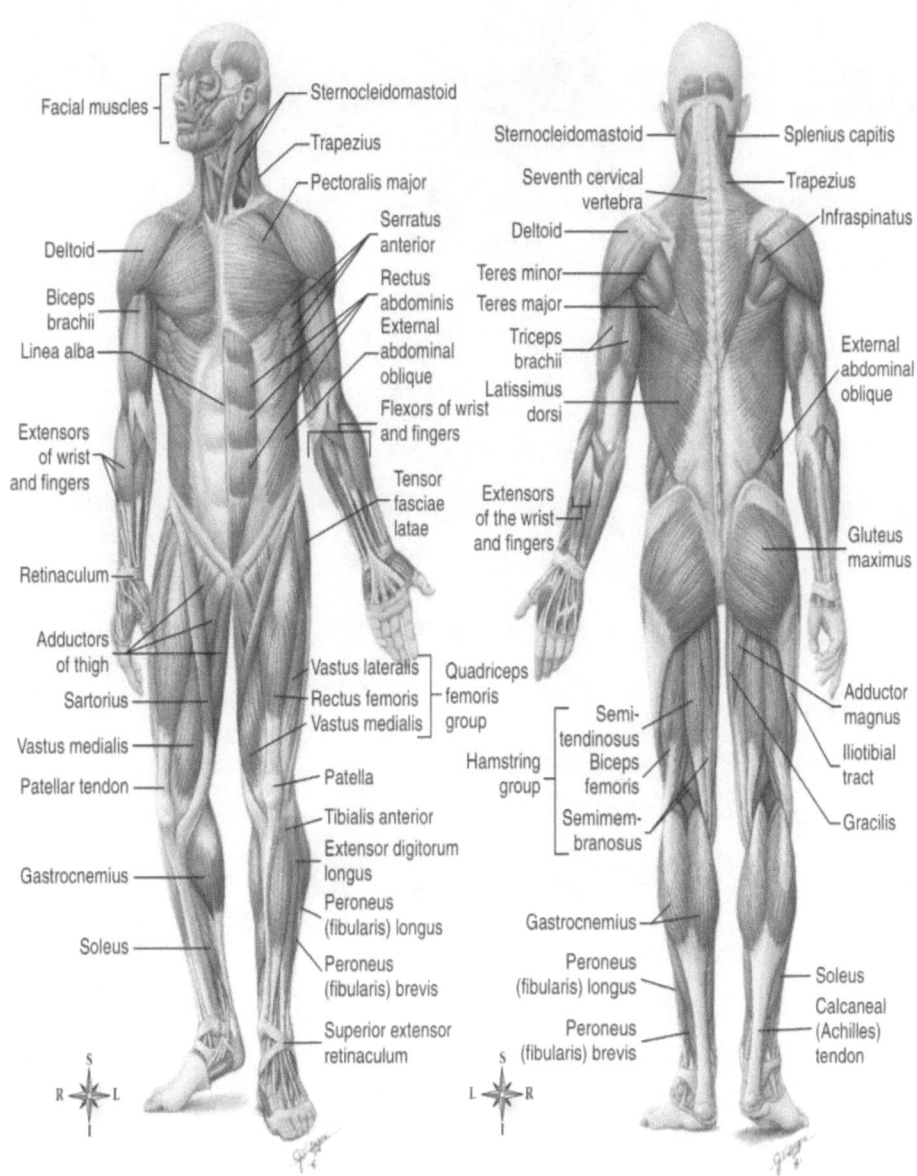

FIGURE 2-30 Body Musculature, Anterior View.   **FIGURE 2-31 Body Musculature, Posterior View.**

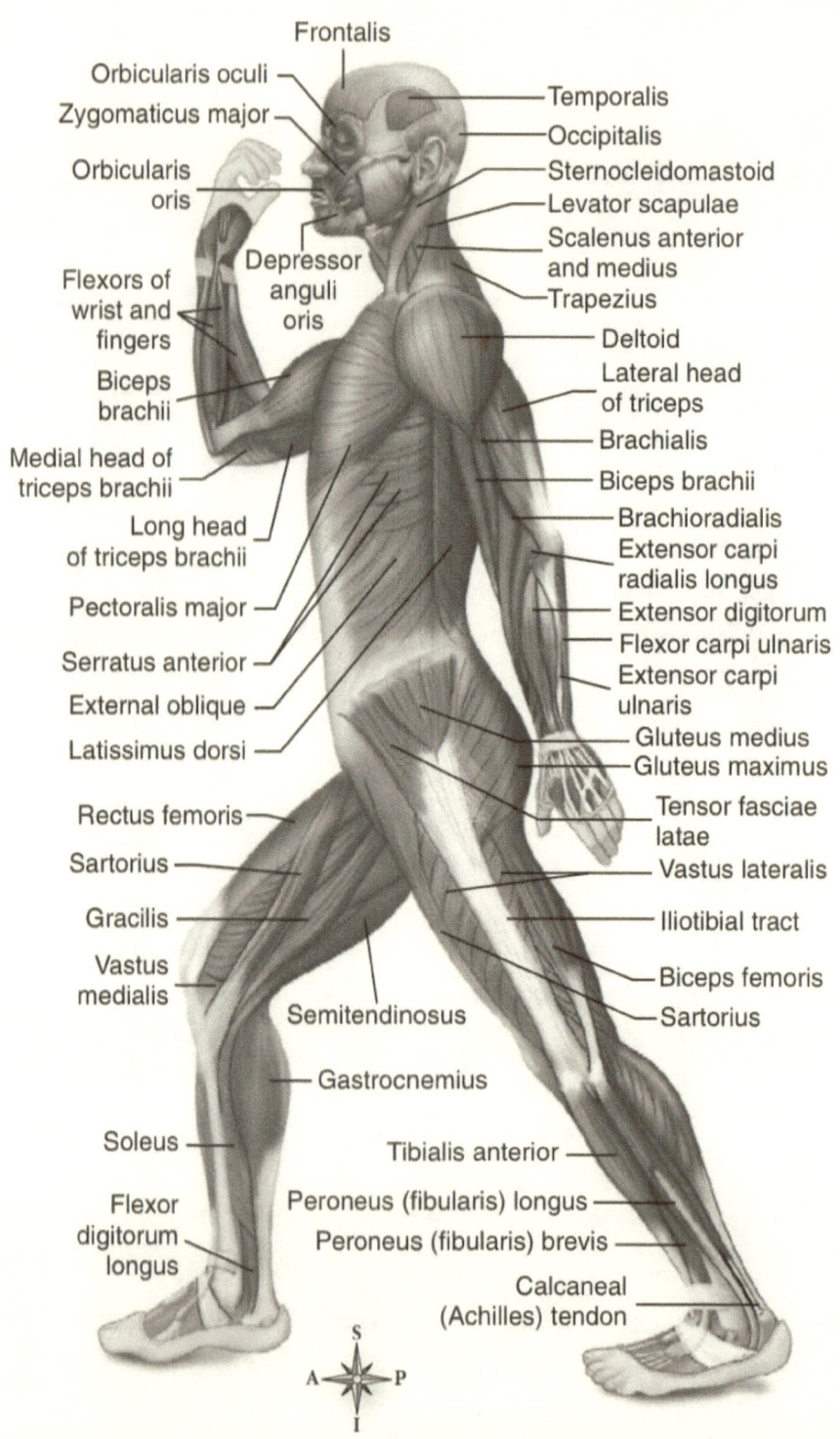

Frontalis

Orbicularis oculi

Zygomaticus major

Orbicularis
oris

Flexors of
wrist and
fingers

Biceps
brachii

Medial head of
triceps brachii

Long head
of triceps brachii

Pectoralis major

Serratus anterior

External oblique

Latissimus dorsi

Rectus femoris

Sartorius

Gracilis

Vastus
medialis

Soleus

Flexor
digitorum
longus

Depressor
anguli
oris

Semitendinosus

Gastrocnemius

Temporalis

Occipitalis

Sternocleidomastoid

Levator scapulae

Scalenus anterior
and medius

Trapezius

Deltoid

Lateral head
of triceps

Brachialis

Biceps brachii

Brachioradialis

Extensor carpi
radialis longus

Extensor digitorum

Flexor carpi ulnaris

Extensor carpi
ulnaris

Gluteus medius

Gluteus maximus

Tensor fasciae
latae

Vastus lateralis

Iliotibial tract

Biceps femoris

Sartorius

Tibialis anterior

Peroneus (fibularis) longus

Peroneus (fibularis) brevis

Calcaneal
(Achilles) tendon

S

A ✧ P

I

FIGURE 2-32 Body Musculature, Lateral View.

<u>Spine</u>

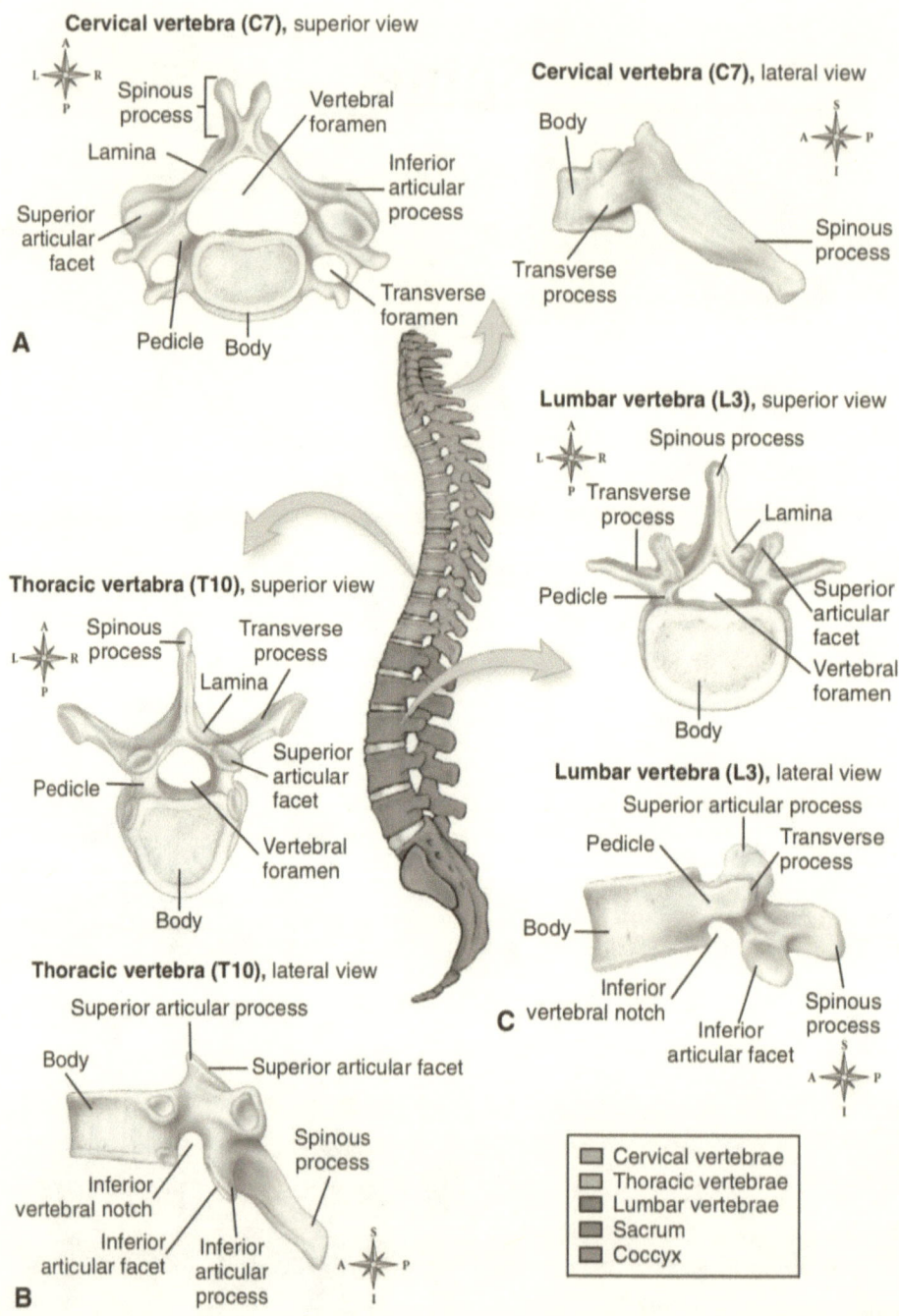

Cervical vertebra (C7), superior view

Spinous process
Vertebral foramen
Lamina
Inferior articular process
Superior articular facet
Pedicle
Body
Transverse foramen

A

Cervical vertebra (C7), lateral view

Body
Spinous process
Transverse process

Thoracic vertabra (T10), superior view

Spinous process
Transverse process
Lamina
Pedicle
Superior articular facet
Vertebral foramen
Body

Thoracic vertebra (T10), lateral view

Superior articular process
Body
Superior articular facet
Spinous process
Inferior vertebral notch
Inferior articular facet
Inferior articular process

B

Lumbar vertebra (L3), superior view

Spinous process
Transverse process
Lamina
Pedicle
Superior articular facet
Vertebral foramen
Body

Lumbar vertebra (L3), lateral view

Superior articular process
Pedicle
Transverse process
Body
Inferior vertebral notch
Inferior articular facet
Spinous process

C

Cervical vertebrae
Thoracic vertebrae
Lumbar vertebrae
Sacrum
Coccyx

- 48 -

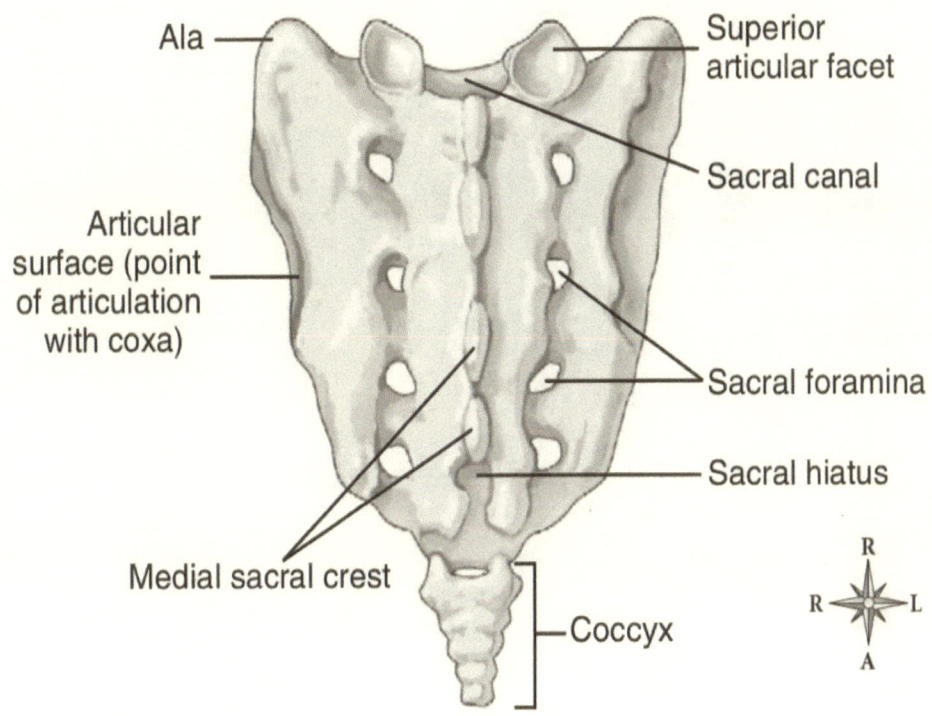

Ala

Superior
articular facet

Sacral canal

Articular
surface (point
of articulation
with coxa)

Sacral foramina

Sacral hiatus

Medial sacral crest

Coccyx

R

R — L

A

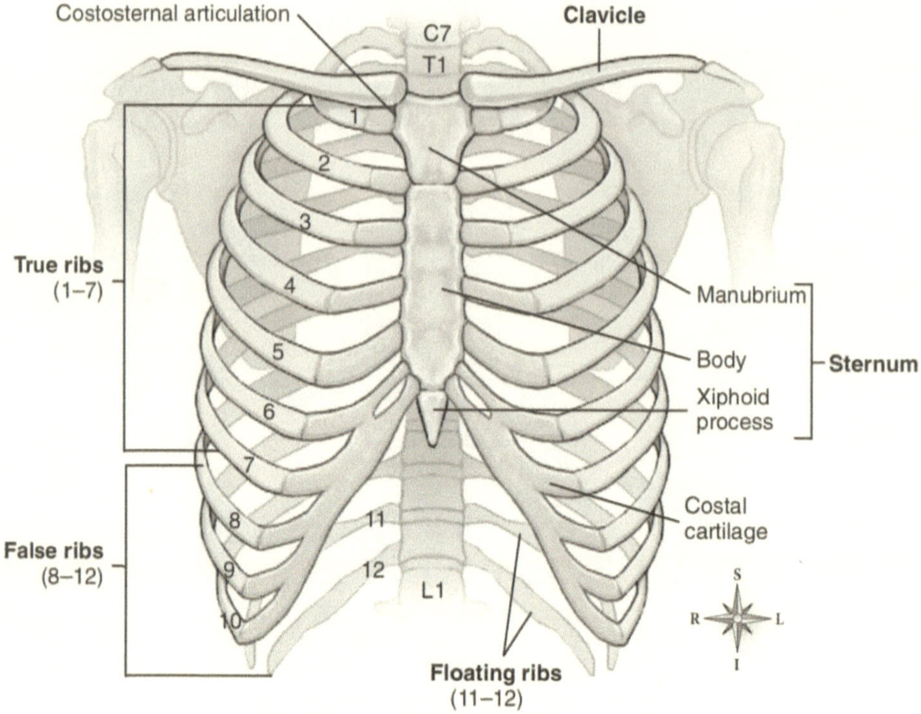

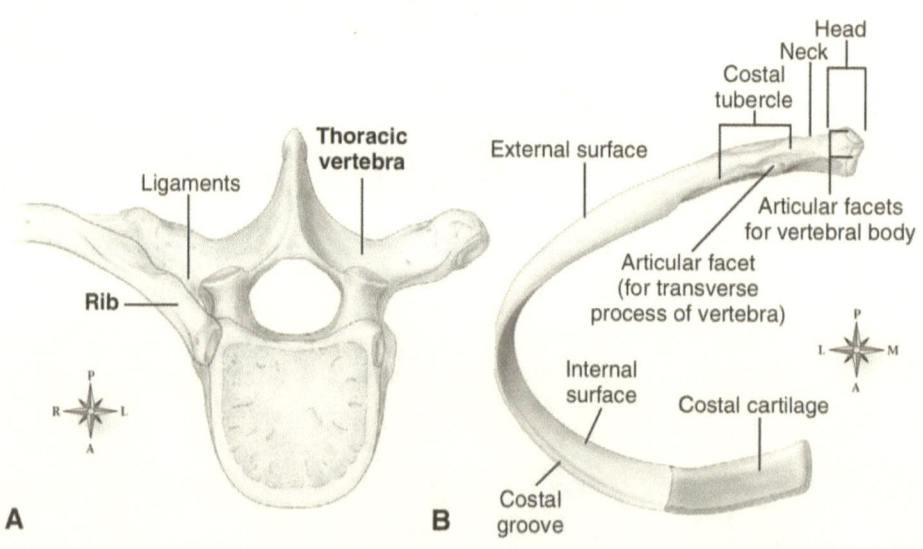

Costosternal articulation

Clavicle

C7
T1

True ribs
(1–7)

1
2
3
4
5
6
7
8
9
10
11
12

Manubrium

Body

Xiphoid
process

Sternum

Costal
cartilage

False ribs
(8–12)

L1

S
R — L
I

Floating ribs
(11–12)

FIGURE 2-16 Thoracic (Rib) Cage and Clavicle.

Head
Neck
Costal
tubercle

Ligaments

Thoracic
vertebra

External surface

Rib

Articular facets
for vertebral body

Articular facet
(for transverse
process of vertebra)

Internal
surface

Costal cartilage

Costal
groove

P
R — L
A

P
L — M
A

A

B

FIGURE 2-17 Rib. **A,** Articulation of rib and vertebra. **B,** Structure of left fifth rib.

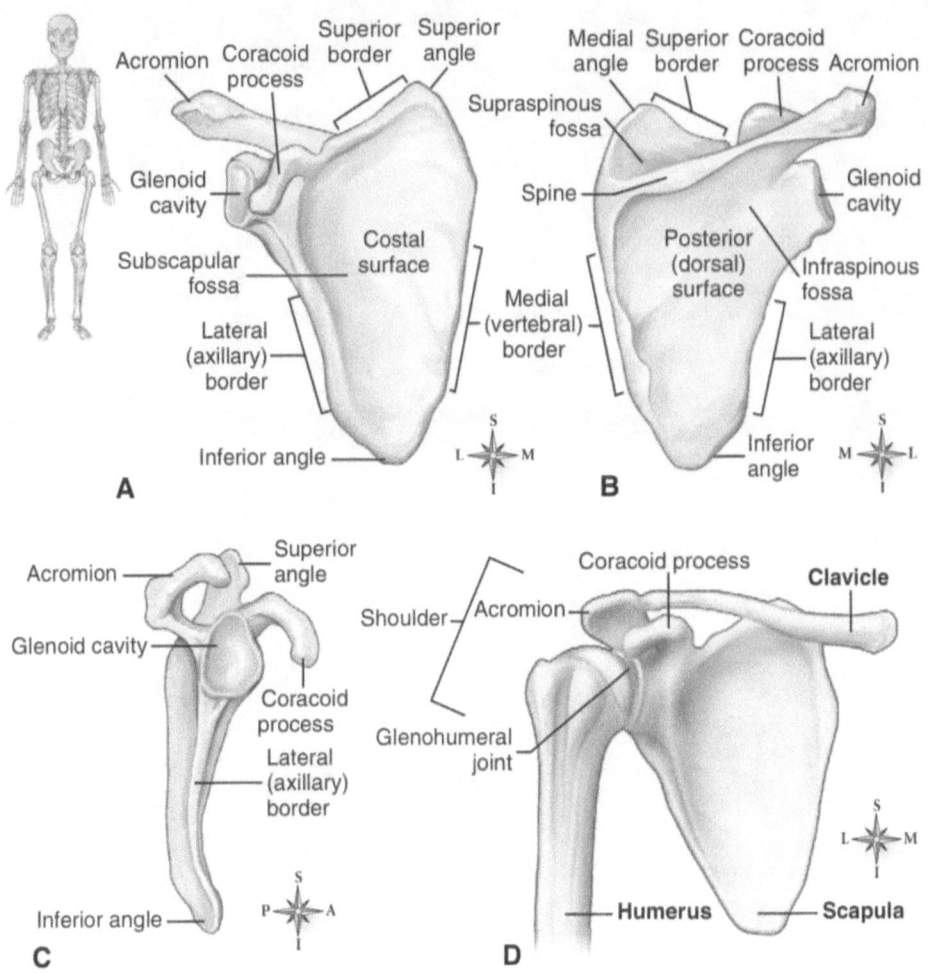

FIGURE 2-18 Right Scapula.
A, Anterior view.
B, Posterior view.
C, Lateral view.
D, Posterior view showing articulation with clavicle.

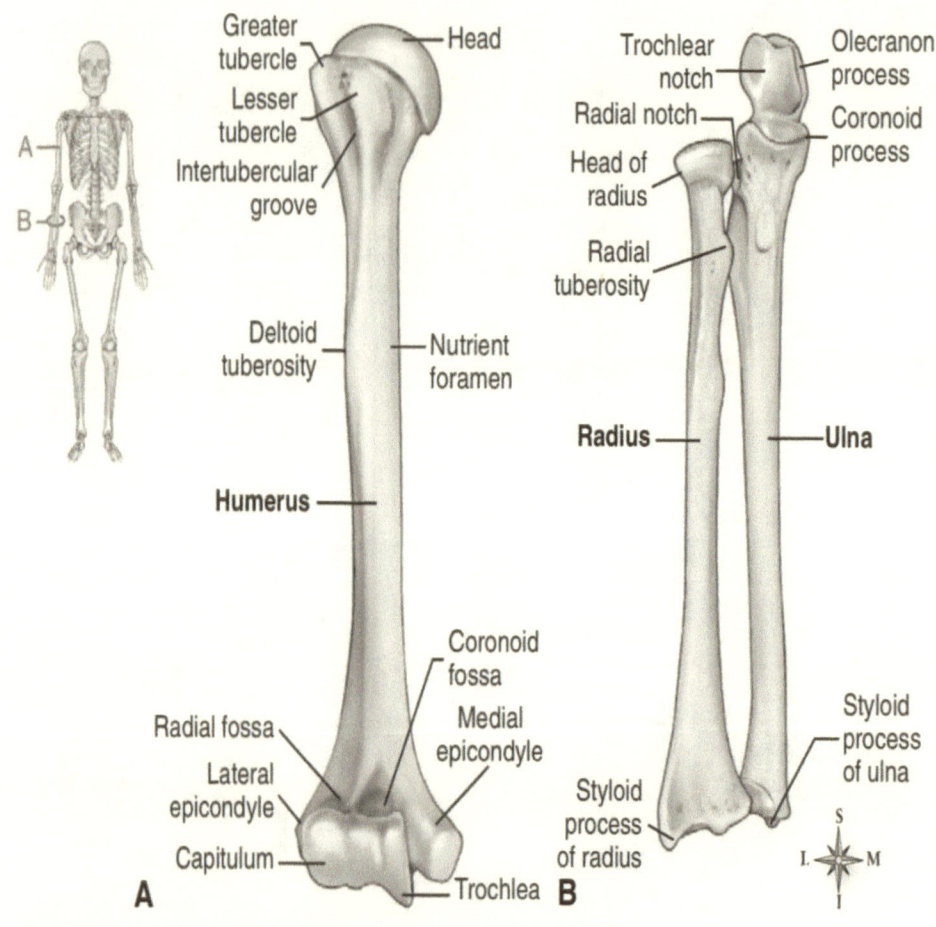

FIGURE 2-19 Bones of the Right Arm and Forearm, Anterior View.
A, Humerus (arm). **B,** Radius and ulna (forearm).

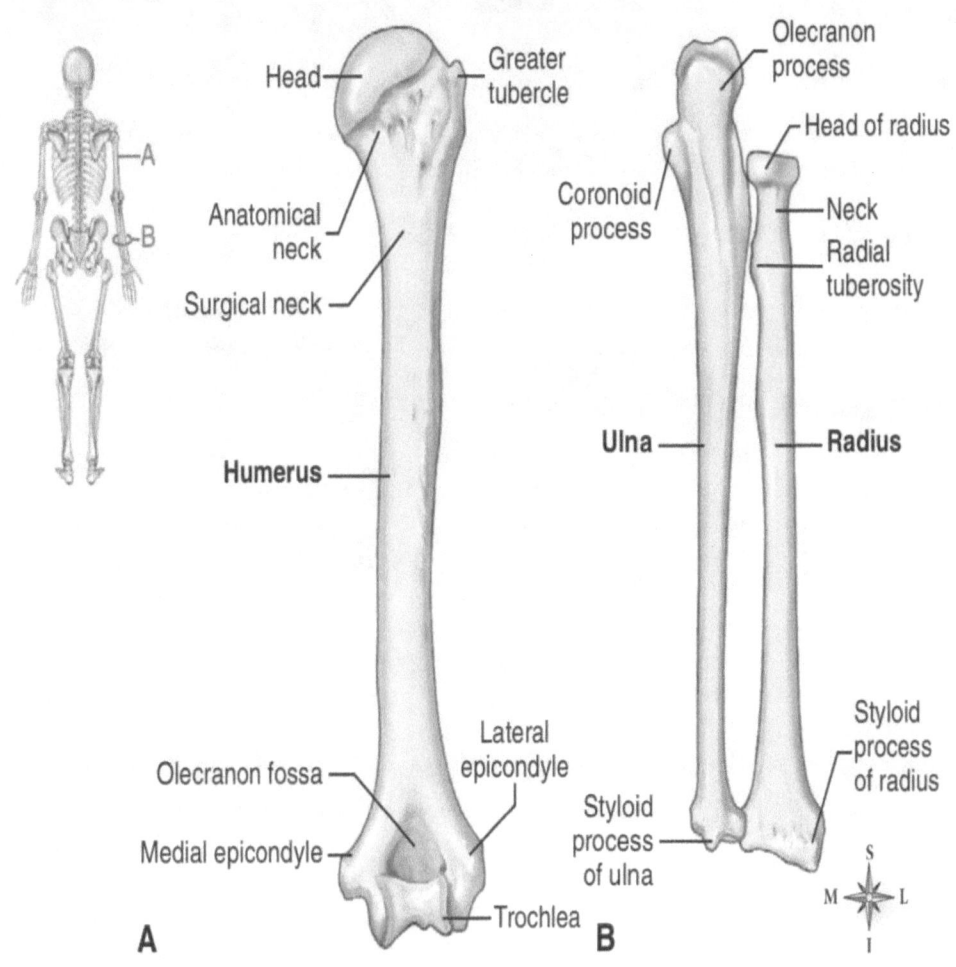

Head — Greater tubercle

Anatomical neck

Surgical neck

Humerus —

Olecranon fossa —

Medial epicondyle —

Lateral epicondyle

Trochlea

A

Olecranon process

Coronoid process

Head of radius

Neck

Radial tuberosity

Ulna — — Radius

Styloid process of radius

Styloid process of ulna

B

S
M — L
I

FIGURE 2-20 Bones of the Right Arm, Posterior View.
A, Humerus (arm). **B,** Radius and ulna (forearm).

Bones and Markings	Pronunciations	Translations	Descriptions and Hints
Clavicle	KLAV-i-kul	Little key or bolt	Collar bones; the shoulder girdle is joined to the axial skeleton by the articulation of the clavicles with the sternum (the scapula does not form a joint with the axial skeleton)
Sternal end	STER-nel end	End near sternum	Thick end near the sternum
Acromial end	ah-KRO-mee-al end	End near acromion (of scapula)	Oval end near the acromion of the scapula
Body (shaft)	BOD-ee (shaft)	Main part (long cylinder)	Central shaft
Scapula	SKAP-yoo-lah	Shoulder	Shoulder blades; the scapulae and clavicles together make up the shoulder girdle
Borders			
Superior border	soo-PEER-ee-or BOHR-der	Upper	Upper margin
Medial (vertebral) border	MEE-dee-al (VER-teh-bral or ver-TEE-bral) BOHR-der	Middle	Margin toward the vertebral column
Lateral (axillary) border	LAT-er-al (AK-sil-lair-ee) BOHR-der	Side (armpit)	Lateral margin, toward the axilla
Angles	ANG-gulz	Corners	The three corners of the scapula
Inferior angle	in-FEER-ee-or ANG-gul	Lower corner	Corner where the lateral and medial borders meet at the bottom of the scapula
Lateral angle	LAT-er-al ANG-gul	Side corner	Corner where the lateral and superior borders meet at the glenoid cavity
Superior (medial) angle	soo-PEER-ee-or (MEE-dee-al) ANG-gul	Upper (middle) corner	Corner where the medial and superior borders meet at the top of the scapula
Spine	spyne	Thorn	Sharp ridge that runs diagonally across the posterior surface of the shoulder blade
Acromion	ah-KRO-mee-un	Shoulder extremity	Slightly flaring projection at the lateral end of the scapular spine; may be felt at the tip of the shoulder; articulates with the clavicle

Bones and Markings	Pronunciations	Translations	Descriptions and Hints
Coracoid process	KOH-rah-koyd PRAH-ses	Projection like a crow (beak)	Projection on the anterior surface from the upper border of the bone; may be felt in the groove between the deltoid and pectoralis major muscles, about 1 inch below the clavicle
Supraspinous fossa	soo-pra-SPY-nus FOSS-ah	Depression above the spine	Concavity formed above the spine's attachment to the body of the scapula
Infraspinous fossa	in-fra-SPY-nus FOSS-ah	Depression below the spine	Concavity formed below the spine's attachment to the body of the scapula
Subscapular fossa	sub-SKAP-yoo-lar FOSS-ah	Depression below the scapula	Concave surface on the "underside" of the scapula against the rib cage
Glenoid cavity	GLEE-noyd KAV-i-tee	Hollow like an eye socket	Arm socket
Humerus	HYOO-mer-us	Arm	Long bone of the arm
Head	hed	Head	Smooth, hemispherical enlargement at the proximal end of the humerus
Anatomical neck	an-ah-TOM-i-kal nek	Structural narrowing below the head	Oblique groove just below the head
Greater tubercle	GRAYT-er TOO-ber-kul	Larger little bump	Rounded projection lateral to the head on the anterior surface
Lesser tubercle	LESS-er TOO-ber-kul	Smaller little bump	Prominent projection on the anterior surface just below the anatomical neck
Intertubercular groove (sulcus)	in-ter-too-BER-kyool-ar groov (SUL-kus)	Groove between little bumps	Deep groove between the greater and lesser tubercles; the long tendon of the biceps muscle lodges here
Surgical neck	SERJ-ik-al nek	Narrowing below head of clinical interest	Region just below the tubercles; so named because of its liability to fracture

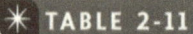 **TABLE 2-11** Upper Extremity Bones and Their Markings—cont'd

Bones and Markings	Pronunciations	Translations	Descriptions and Hints
Deltoid tuberosity	DEL-toyd too-ber-AH-sih-tee	Delta (Δ)-like bump	V-shaped, rough area about midway down the shaft where the deltoid muscle inserts
Radial groove (sulcus)	RAY-dee-al groov (SUL-kus)	Groove related to the radius	Groove that runs obliquely downward from the deltoid tuberosity; lodges the radial nerve
Lateral epicondyle	LAT-er-al ep-i-KON-dyle	Side knuckle-end	Rough projections at the lateral side of the distal end
Medial epicondyle	MEE-dee-al ep-i-KON-dyle	Middle knuckle-end	Rough projections at the medial side of the distal end
Capitulum	kah-PITCH-uh-lum	Little head	Rounded knob below the lateral epicondyle; articulates with the radius; sometimes called the *radial head of the humerus*
Trochlea	TROK-lee-ah	Pulley	Projection with a deep depression through the center, similar to the shape of a pulley; articulates with the ulna
Olecranon fossa	oh-LEK-rah-non FOSS-ah	Ditch for the head (cranium) of elbow	Depression on the posterior surface just above the trochlea; receives the olecranon of the ulna when the forearm extends
Coronoid fossa	KOR-uh-noyd FOSS-ah	Ditch for the crownlike (process)	Depression on the anterior surface above the trochlea; receives the coronoid process of the ulna during flexion of the forearm
Body (shaft)	BOD-ee (shaft)	Main part (long cylinder)	Central shaft
Radius	RAY-dee-us	Staff or spoke	Bone of the thumb side of the forearm
Head	hed	Head	Disk-shaped process that forms the proximal end of the radius; articulates with the capitulum of the humerus and with the radial notch of the ulna
Neck	nek	Neck	Narrowing just distal to the head

Bones and Markings	Pronunciations	Translations	Descriptions and Hints
Phalanges (*sing.,* **phalanx**)	fah-LAN-jeez (fah-LANKS)	Ranks of soldiers	Miniature long bones of the fingers; there are three in each finger and two in each thumb; numbered from the medial/thumb side; each has a *base,* a *shaft,* and a *head;* lined up like a military parade formation
Proximal (I, II, III, IV, V)	PROK-si-mal	Near (Roman 1, 2, 3, 4, 5)	
Middle (II, III, IV, V)	MID-dul	Middle (Roman 2, 3, 4, 5)	
Distal (I, II, III, IV, V)	DIS-tal	Distant (Roman 1, 2, 3, 4, 5)	

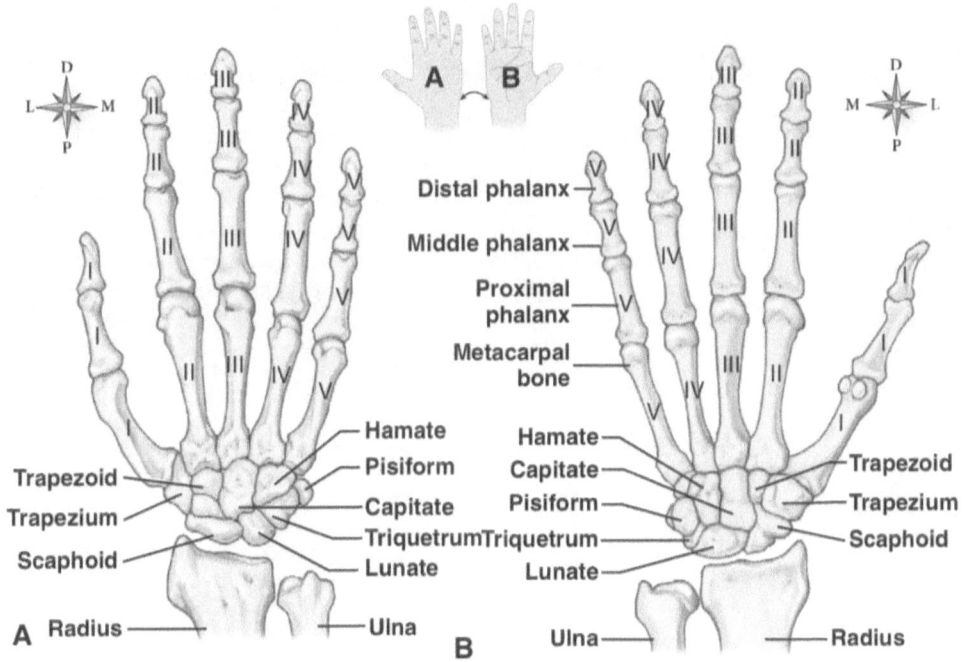

FIGURE 2-21 Bones of the Hand and Wrist.
A, Palmar view of the right hand and wrist.
B, Dorsal view of the right hand and wrist.

Bones and Markings	Pronunciations	Translations	Descriptions and Hints
Radial tuberosity	RAY-dee-al too-ber-AH-sih-tee	Bump of the staff (radius)	Roughened projection on the ulnar side, a short distance below the head; the biceps muscle inserts here
Styloid process	STY-loyd PRAH-ses	Styluslike projection	Protuberance at the distal end on the lateral surface (with the forearm in the anatomical position)
Body (shaft)	BOD-ee (shaft)	Main part (long cylinder)	Central shaft
Ulna	UL-nah	Elbow	Bone of the little finger side of the forearm; longer than the radius
Olecranon	oh-LEK-rah-non	Head (cranium) of elbow	Scooplike process that joins the trochlea of the humerus at the elbow
Coronoid process	KOR-uh-noyd PRAH-ses	Crownlike projection	Projection on the anterior surface of the proximal end of the ulna; the trochlea of the humerus fits snugly between the olecranon and the coronoid processes
Trochlear notch	TROK-lee-ar notch	V-cut for the pulley	Curved notch between the olecranon and the coronoid process into which the trochlea fits; also called the *semilunar notch*
Radial notch	RAY-dee-al notch	V-cut for the staff (radius)	Curved notch that is lateral and inferior to the trochlear (semilunar) notch; the head of the radius fits into this concavity
Head	hed	Head	Rounded process at the distal end; does not articulate with the wrist bones but rather with the fibrocartilaginous disk
Styloid process	STY-loyd PRAH-ses	Projection	Sharp protuberance at the distal end; can be seen from outside on the posterior surface
Carpal bones	KAR-pal bohnz	Bones of wrist	Wrist bones; arranged in two rows (proximal and distal) at the proximal end of the hand

Bones and Markings	Pronunciations	Translations	Descriptions and Hints
Pisiform (lentiform)	PY-zi-form (LEN-ti-form)	Pea-shaped (lens-shaped)	First (medial/thumbside) bone of the proximal row; looks like a slightly flattened pea sticking out from the triquetrum on the palmar side
Triquetrum (triangular, cuneiform, or pyramidal)	try-KWET-rum or try-KWEET-rum (try-ANG-yoo-lar, KYOO-neh-form, or pih-RAM-id-al)	Three-cornered (three-angled, wedge-shaped, or pyramidlike)	Second bone of the proximal row; looks like a triangle from the dorsal view; only bone connected to the pisiform
Lunate (semilunar)	LOON-ayt (sem-ee-LOON-er)	Moonlike (half-moon–like)	Third bone of the proximal row; its crescent outline resembles a half moon
Scaphoid (navicular)	SKAF-oyd (na-VIK-yoo-lar)	Boat-shaped	Fourth bone of the proximal row; the curving largest bone of the row; resembles a small boat
Hamate (unciform)	HAY-mayt or HAM-ayt (UN-si-form)	Hook-shaped	First (medial/thumbside) bone of the distal row; wedgelike bone has large "hook" on the palmar side; dorsal outline resembles a ham
Capitate	KAP-ee-tayt or KAP-i-tayt	Having a head	Second bone of the distal row; largest of all of the carpals; has a "head" that fits into the curve of the scaphoid and the lunate
Trapezoid (lesser multangular)	TRAP-eh-zoyd (LESS-er mul-TANG-yoo-lar)	Tablelike (smaller many-angled)	Third bone of the distal row; smallest bone of the row; wedge-like, pointing toward the palmar side
Trapezium (greater multangular)	tra-PEEZ-ee-um (GRAYT-er mul-TANG-yoo-lar)	Table (larger many-angled)	Fourth bone of the distal row; trapezoid outline with a deep groove on the palmar side
Metacarpal bones	met-ah-KAR-pal bohnz	Bones after the wrist	Long bones that form the supporting framework of the palm of the hand; numbered from the medial (thumb) side; each has a *base*, a *shaft*, and a *head*
I	won	Roman 1	
II	too	Roman 2	
III	three	Roman 3	
IV	fohr	Roman 4	
V	fyve	Roman 5	

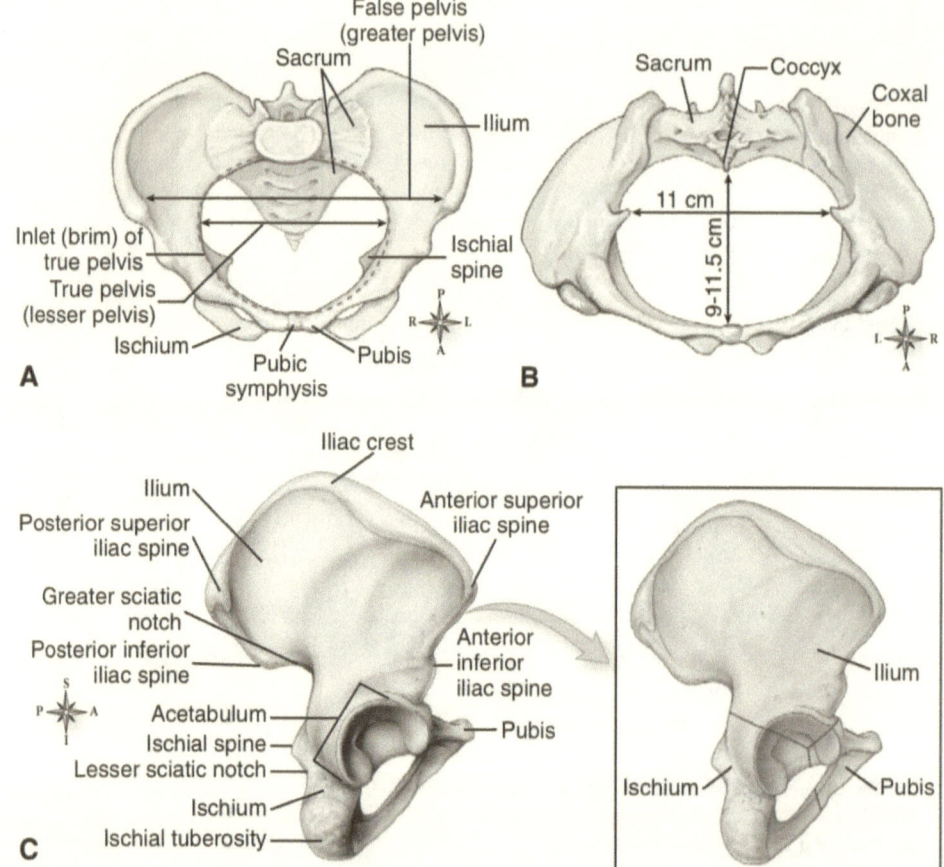

FIGURE 2-22 Pelvic Girdle. The **pelvic girdle** *(pelvis)* is a ring of three bones: the sacrum and both pelvic bones.

A, Superior view. Note that the brim of the true pelvis *(dotted line)* marks the boundary between the superior false pelvis *(pelvis major)* and the inferior true pelvis *(pelvis minor)*.

B, Posterior view.

C, Lateral view of the right pelvic bone. The inset shows major divisions.

A comparison of the male and female pelvises is shown in Figure 2-25.

Bones and Markings	Pronunciations	Translations	Descriptions and Hints
Coxal bone (pelvic bone or coxa)	KOK-sal bohn (PEL-vik bohn or KOK-sah)	Hip bone (basin bone or hip)	Large hip bone (pelvic bone); with the sacrum and the coccyx, forms the basinlike pelvic cavity; lower extremities are attached to the axial skeleton by the coxal bones
Ilium	IL-ee-um	Flank	Upper, flaring portion (this is a separate bone during early development)
Ischium	ISS-kee-um	Hip joint	Lower, posterior portion (this is a separate bone during early development)
Pubis (pl., pubes)	PYOO-bis (PYOO-beez)	Groin	Medial, anterior section (this is a separate bone during early development)
Acetabulum	ass-eh-TAB-yoo-lum	Vinegar cup	Hip socket; formed by the union of the ilium, the ischium, and the pubis
Iliac crest	IL-ee-ak krest	Flank ridges	Upper, curving boundary of the ilium
Iliac spines	IL-ee-ak spynez	Flank thorns	Sharp projections at the "corners" of the ilium
Anterior superior spine	an-TEER-ee-or soo-PEER-ee-or spyne	Front upper thorn	Prominent projection at the anterior end of the iliac crest; can be felt externally as the "point" of the hip
Anterior inferior spine	an-TEER-ee-or in-FEER-ee-or spyne	Front lower thorn	Less prominent projection a short distance below the anterior superior spine
Posterior superior spine	pohs-TEER-ee-or soo-PEER-ee-or spyne	Back upper thorn	At the posterior end of the iliac crest
Posterior inferior spine	pohs-TEER-ee-or in-FEER-ee-or spyne	Back lower thorn	Just below the posterior superior spine
Greater sciatic notch	GRAYT-er sye-AT-ik notch	Larger V-cut of hip	Large notch on the posterior surface of the ilium just below the posterior inferior spine
Ischial tuberosity	ISS-kee-al too-ber-AH-sih-tee	Hip bump	Large, rough, quadrilateral process that forms the inferior part of the ischium; in an erect sitting position, the body

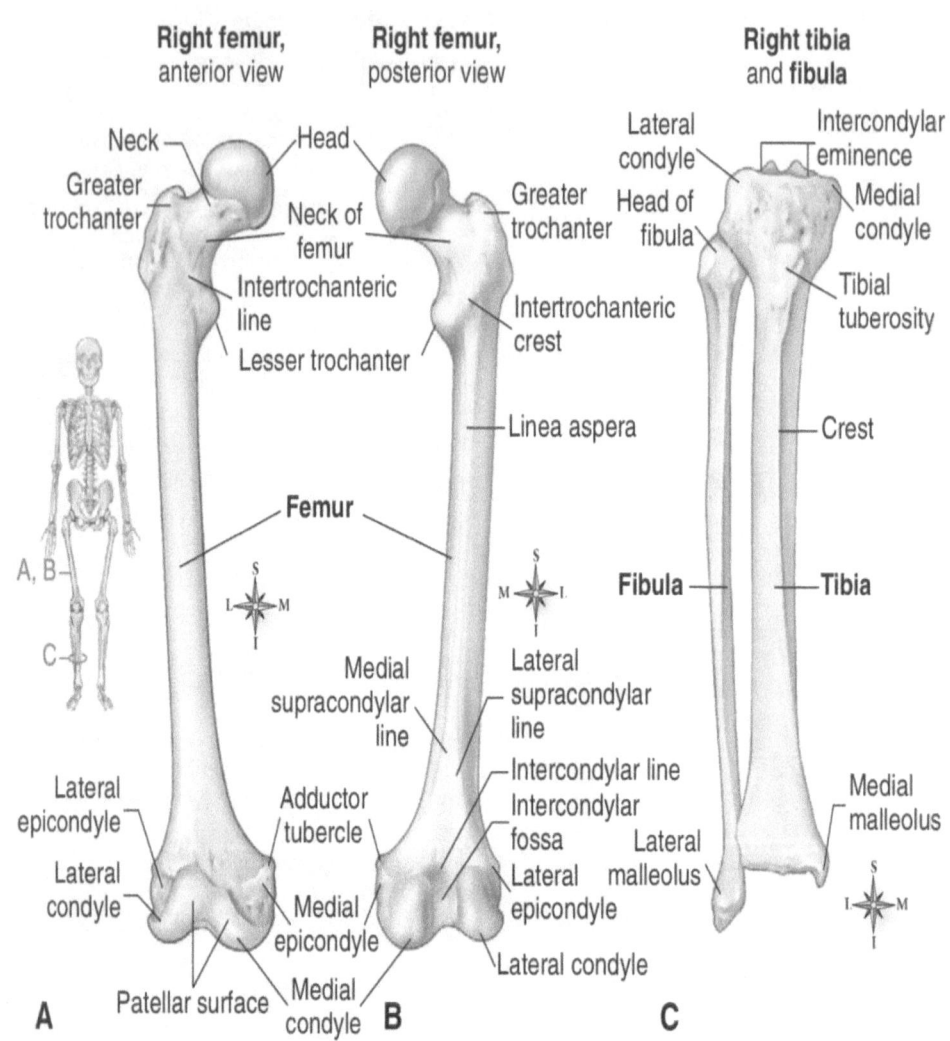

FIGURE 2-23 Bones of the Thigh and Leg.
A, Right femur, anterior surface.
B, Right femur, posterior surface.
C, Right tibia and fibula, anterior surface.

Bones and Markings	Pronunciations	Translations	Descriptions and Hints
True pelvis (or greater pelvis)	troo PEL-vis (GRAYT-er PEL-vis)	True basin	Space below the pelvic brim; true "basin," with bone and muscle walls and a muscle floor; the pelvic organs are located in this space
False pelvis (or lesser pelvis)	fals PEL-vis (LESS-er PEL-vis)	False basin	Broad, shallow space above the pelvic brim or the pelvic inlet; the name "false pelvis" is misleading, because this space is actually part of the abdominal cavity rather than the pelvic cavity
Pelvic outlet	PEL-vik OWT-let	Exit of basin (drain)	Irregular circumference that marks the lower limits of the true pelvis; bounded by the tip of the coccyx and two ischial tuberosities
Pelvic girdle (or bony pelvis)	PEL-vik GERD-ul (BOHN-ee PEL-vis)	Basinlike belt	Complete bony ring; composed of two coxal (pelvic) bones, the sacrum, and the coccyx; forms a firm base by which the trunk rests on the thighs and for the attachment of the lower extremities to the axial skeleton
Femur	FEE-mur		Thigh bone; the largest, strongest bone of the body
Head	hed	Head	Rounded upper end of the bone; fits into the acetabulum
Neck	nek	Narrowing below the head	Constricted portion just below the head
Greater trochanter	GRAYT-er troh-KAN-ter (or TROH-kan-ter)	Bigger runner	Protuberance located inferiorly and laterally to the head
Lesser trochanter	LESS-er troh-KAN-ter (or TROH-kan-ter)	Smaller runner	Small protuberance located inferiorly and medially to the greater trochanter
Intertrochanteric line	in-ter-troh-KAN-ter-ik lyne	Line between runners	Line that extends between the greater and lesser trochanter
Linea aspera	LEEN-ee-ah (or LIN-ee-ah) ASS-per-ah	Rough line	Prominent ridge that extends lengthwise along the concave posterior surface

Bones and Markings	Pronunciations	Translations	Descriptions and Hints
Supracondylar lines (ridges)	soo-prah-KON-dil-er lynz (RIJ-ez)	Above-knuckle ridges	Two ridges formed by the division of the linea aspera at its lower end; the medial supracondylar ridge extends inward to the inner condyle and the lateral ridge to the outer condyle
Medial condyle	MEE-dee-al KON-dyle	Middle knuckle	Large, rounded bulge at the distal end of the femur; on the medial aspect
Lateral condyle	LAT-er-al KON-dyle	Side knuckle	Large, rounded bulge at the distal end of the femur; on the lateral aspect
Medial epicondyle	MEE-dee-al ep-i-KON-dyle	Middle knuckle-end	Blunt projection from the side of the medial condyle
Lateral epicondyle	LAT-er-al ep-i-KON-dyle	Side knuckle-end	Blunt projection from the side of the lateral condyle
Adductor tubercle	ad-DUK-ter TOO-ber-kul	Small bump of the bringer-in (muscles)	Small projection just above the medial condyle; marks the termination of the medial supracondylar ridge
Trochlea	TROK-lee-ah	Pulley	Smooth depression between the condyles on the anterior surface; articulates with the patella
Intercondylar fossa (notch)	in-trah-KON-dil-er FOSS-ah (notch)	Between-knuckle ditch	Deep depression between the condyles on the posterior surface; the cruciate ligaments, which help to bind the femur to the tibia, lodge in this notch
Body (shaft)	BOD-ee (shaft)	Main part (long cylinder)	Central shaft
Intertrochanteric crest	in-ter-troh-kan-TAYR-ik krest	Ridge between trochanters (large bumps)	Raised ridge on the posterior surface that runs between the greater and lesser trochanter
Intercondylar line	in-ter-KON-dil-er lyne	Line between knuckles	Ridge on the posterior surface between the bases of the condyles
Patella	pah-TEL-ah	Little pan (kneecap)	Kneecap; the largest sesamoid bone of the body; embedded in the tendon of the quadriceps femoris muscle
Tibia	TIB-ee-ah	Shinbone	Shin bone

Bones and Markings	Pronunciations	Translations	Descriptions and Hints
Medial condyle	MEE-dee-al KON-dyle	Middle knuckle	Bulging medial prominence at the proximal end of the tibia; the surface is concave for articulation with the femur
Lateral condyle	LAT-er-al KON-dyle	Side knuckle	Concave prominence lateral to the medial condyle
Intercondylar eminence	in-ter-KON-dil-er EM-in-ents	Raised thing between knuckles	Upward projection on the articular surface between the condyles
Crest	krest	Ridge (comb)	Sharp ridge on the anterior surface
Tibial tuberosity	TIB-ee-al too-ber-AH-sih-tee	Bump of the shinbone	Projection in the midline on the anterior surface
Medial malleolus (pl., malleoli)	MEE-dee-al MAL-lee-o-lus	Little hammer toward the middle	Rounded downward projection at the distal end of the tibia; forms the prominence on the medial surface of the ankle
Body (shaft)	BOD-ee (shaft)	Main part (long cylinder)	Central shaft
Fibula	FIB-yoo-lah	Clasp	Long, slender bone of the lateral side of the leg
Head	hed	Head	Proximal enlargement
Neck	nek	Narrowing below the head	Constricted portion just below the head
Lateral malleolus (pl., malleoli)	LAT-er-al MAL-lee-o-lus (mal-LEE-o-lee or mal-LEE-o-lye)	Little hammer to the side	Rounded prominence at the distal end of the fibula; forms the prominence on the lateral surface of the ankle
Body (shaft)	BOD-ee (shaft)	Main part (long cylinder)	Central shaft
Tarsal bones	TAR-sal bohnz	Ankle bones	Bones that form the heel and proximal or posterior half of the foot
Calcaneus	kal-KAY-nee-us	Heel bone	Heel bone
Talus	TAY-lus	Anklebone or knucklebone	Uppermost of the tarsal bones; articulates with the tibia and the fibula; boxed between the medial and lateral malleoli
Navicular (scaphoid)	na-VIK-yoo-lar (SKAF-oyd)	Boat-shaped	Curved bone anterior and slightly medial to talus and posterior to the cuneiform bones; looks like a little boat

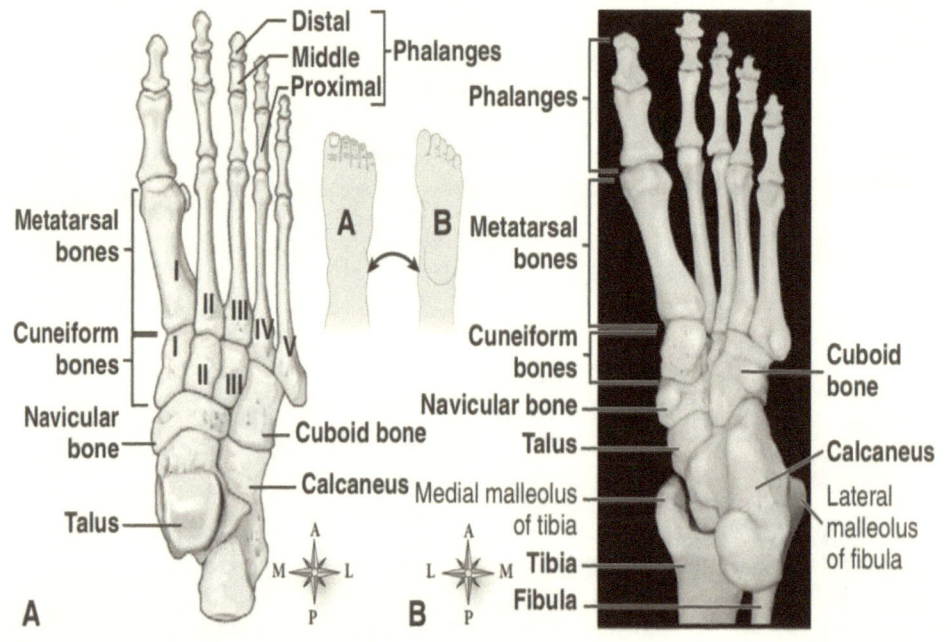

FIGURE 2-24 The Foot.
A, Superior view.
B, Inferior view.

Lower Extremity Bones and Their Markings—cont'd

Bones and Markings	Pronunciations	Translations	Descriptions and Hints
Cuboid	KYOO-boyd	Like a cube	Looks like a cube from the top but really more of a pyramid (the base is medial); on the lateral side of the foot, anterior to the calcaneus and posterior to metatarsals IV and V
Medial cuneiform (I)	MEE-dee-al KYOO-neh-form	Wedge-shaped (bone) toward the middle (Roman 1)	Looks like a cube from the top but really more of a wedge; between navicular and metatarsal I
Intermediate cuneiform (II)	in-ter-MEE-dee-it KYOO-neh-form	Wedge-shaped (bone) in the middle (Roman 2)	Looks like a cube from the top but really more of a wedge; between navicular and metatarsal II
Lateral cuneiform (III)	LAT-er-al KYOO-neh-form	Wedge-shaped (bone) to the side (Roman 3)	Looks like a cube from the top but really more of a wedge; between navicular and metatarsal III
Arches of foot	ARCH-ez ov foot	Curves of foot	Curves of the bones of the foot and ankle that, along with muscles and other soft tissues, properly support the mass of the skeleton
Longitudinal arches	lon-jih-TOO-di-nal ARCH-ez	Lengthwise curves	Tarsal and metatarsal bones so arranged as to form an arch from the front to the back of the foot
Medial arch	MEE-dee-al arch	Toward middle	Formed by the calcaneus, the talus, the navicular, the cuneiforms, and three medial metatarsal bones
Lateral arch	LAT-er-al arch	To the side	Formed by the calcaneus, the cuboid, and two lateral metatarsal bones
Transverse (or metatarsal) arch	tranz-VERS (met-ah-TAR-sal) arch	Turned-across (or after-the-ankle) curve	Metatarsal and distal row of tarsal bones (cuneiforms and cuboid) articulated so as to form an arch across the foot; bones are kept in two arched positions by means of powerful ligaments in the sole of the foot and by muscles and tendons

Types of Joints

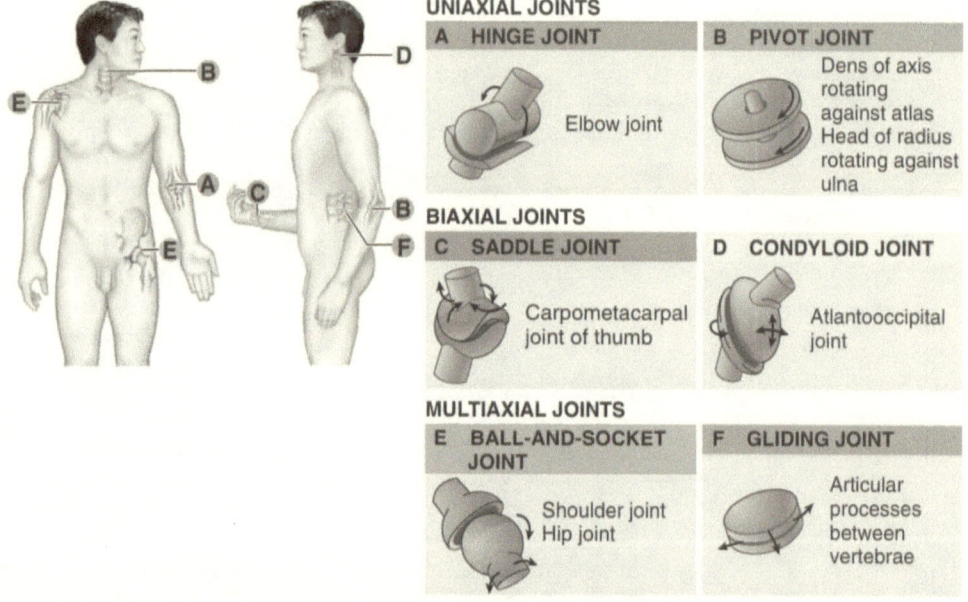

FIGURE 2-29 Types of Synovial Joints. In these simplified cartoons, notice that the shapes of the articulating bones dictate the type of movement that is permitted at each joint.

Classification of Synovial Joints

Types	Examples	Structure	Movement
Uniaxial			*Around one axis; in one place*
Hinge	Elbow joint	Spool-shaped process that fits into a concave socket	Flexion and extension only
Pivot	Joint between the first and second cervical vertebrae	Arch-shaped process that fits around a peglike process	Rotation
Biaxial			*Around two axes that are perpendicular to each other; in two planes*
Saddle	Thumb joint between the first metacarpal and the carpal bone	Saddle-shaped bone that fits into a socket that is concave–convex–concave	Flexion and extension in one plane; abduction and adduction in the other plane; opposing the thumb to the fingers
Condyloid (ellipsoidal)	Joint between the radius and the carpal bones	Oval condyle that fits into an elliptical socket	Flexion and extension in one plane; abduction and adduction in the other plane
Multiaxial			*Around many axes*
Ball and socket	Shoulder joint and hip	Ball-shaped process that fits into a concave socket	Widest range of movement: flexion, extension, abduction, adduction, rotation, and circumduction
Gliding	Joints between the articular facets of adjacent vertebrae; joints between the carpal and tarsal bones	Relatively flat articulating surfaces	Gliding movements without any angular or circular movements

References:

1. Crisologo, C. (2018, May 28). 5 Physical Therapy Settings to Explore Before Applying to PT School • Student Doctor Network.

2. Patton, K. T., Colrus, B., & Kulka, J. (2014). Survival guide for anatomy & physiology: Tips, techniques, and shortcuts for learning about the structure and function of the human body with style, ease, and good humor. St. Louis, MO: Elsevier.